DEDICATION

For my wife.

Alice Fisher is my hero and a true friend. We started a conversation twenty-two years ago and have not stopped talking since.

Thinking back to when I had my stroke and was diagnosed with aphasia, I really didn't know what to do or how I was to get through it. So, Alice took over. Since then, we haven't missed a link. For that and for her, my happiness and gratefulness have grown.

• • •

A special thank you to Mary Beth and McKinley, for without you, this book would not have been possible.

FOREWORD

Dear Jeffrey,

Today you jumped rope. You put the handles in each hand, whipped the rope forward, and hopped when it came around. For most people that might not sound like much, but for you it means freedom, determination, and ten years after your stroke, even more progress.

…'I had never encountered aphasia before, but that didn't stop us. In fact, it only made you stronger.

Over these past couple years as your coach and your friend, I've come to learn so much about this life through our collaboration. If I were to sum it up, it would go like this: Life is a series of events, and we have the opportunity to choose the way we respond to those events. If we choose wisely, our lives will unfold in a miraculous way.

You have the choice to be miraculous. I am proud to know you.

Best,
Coach Alan
Co-Founder and Head Coach, Rhapsody Fitness

NEVER
GIVE UP

A Memoir

JEFFREY FISHER

Cover photo taken by Ed Brantley of Valerie + Ed Photography

Distribution by Bublish, Inc.

ISBN: 978-1-64704-489-3 (paperback)
ISBN: 978-1-64704-490-9 (hardcover)
ISBN: 978-1-64704-488-6 (eBook)

CONTENTS

Part 1 Setting the Stage: Prestroke

Part 2 Key Takeaways

Part 3 Where Jeffrey Is Today and What's Next

Appendix

PART I

SETTING THE STAGE:
PRESTROKE

START HERE

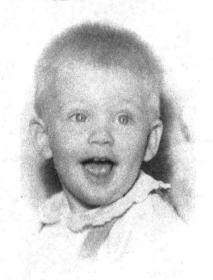

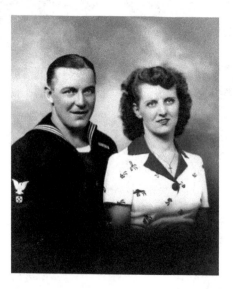

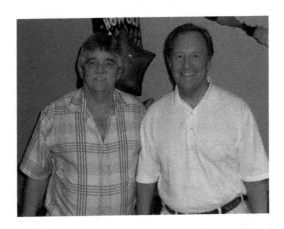

This classic snapshot of an American family starts in Reading, Pennsylvania. A family of four is making their way through life and the world in the 1950s. Jeffrey was born on July 29, 1950, becoming the forever baby of his family.

They were a military family, and Jeffrey's father was a Navy brigadier serving on the USS Brittany as a boatswain mate, tasked with four-year tours and responsible for the upkeep of the ship's external structure.

While the man of the house was away serving his country, Jeffrey's mother, Marian, worked as a candymaker at Bortz in Reading, Pennsylvania, which has since gone out of business. His mother and grandmother were major players in his family in his father's absence.

With a brother six years his senior, Jeffrey was a self-proclaimed spoiled brat—never wrong and always cushioned by his doting Grandmom. While their mother was not as active as Grandmom, Marian did what she was supposed to do as a mother. Moving only twice in their childhood, the Fishers landed at 1142 Locust Street in Reading, Pennsylvania. This row home in the city had a small backyard that was just enough room for young Jeffrey and Jan to explore their imaginary worlds and test their athletic skills.

His older brother, Jan, followed in his father's footsteps to become a die-hard Navy fan. On the other hand, Jeffrey, who was never one to fall in line, rooted for the Army any chance he got. One could chalk this up to sibling rivalry, but it was less of a competition and more of a missed connection. Being six years apart, Jan and Jeffrey seemed to run parallel races, being close enough to keep an eye on the other but far enough away to pave their own paths. Looking back, Jeffrey would say the relationship was honorable—no more, no less.

Jeffrey's father had a drinking problem, which would be what eventually killed him. Despite his affliction, Jeffrey saw his dad as a kind man and industrious worker, who set the example that nothing was given but earned.

Once out of the Navy, Jeffrey's father was present, but not overly active. He worked for the rest of his civilian life as a bartender at the Press Club in Reading. This chosen occupation unfortunately enabled his addiction and was a detriment to his health. He never showed up to school programs or sporting events, but it was never that much of a disappointment to Jeffrey. Back in those days, it did not feel like anyone was too close with their father, so he was never particularly missed. Despite their estrangement, Jeffrey and his father shared a mutually respectful relationship, leaving each other to live and let live.

It was not until Jeffrey was thirteen that he realized his father always had a drink in his hand. Jeffrey was a shy and quiet kid up until this point. When his father's health began to decline, this realization forced Jeffrey to break out of his shell and step into more of a leadership role in the home. Dealing with hardships will do that to you. A short two years after this, Jeffrey's father died.

Their family would never talk about what led to his father drinking himself to death—or at least not to Jeffrey.

At the funeral, Jeffrey's mother took her sons by the arm, looked them square in the eye, and said, "It's just you and me now kids." This recalls the moment as marking the end of his childhood.

After their father died, the Fisher boys were raised by their mother and Grandmom. Jeffrey's mother was as sharp as a tack, who was unwavering and had convinced her boys that she had eyes in the back of her head. Both caring and confident, she continually put Jeffrey on a pedestal.

Grandmom, however, was a wildcard with a boisterous laugh that would shake the walls. She always took Jeffrey's side and defended him, especially when Navy would beat Army. Soon, the Fishers moved to the same street as Grandmom, and the boys enjoyed being just a few houses down from either of their two favorite ladies. These wonder women *had* those boys—together, they were like a sun around which their world orbited.

Jeffrey looks back on these years as times of freedom, exploration, and no questions asked. There were no helicopter moms then. He remembers leaving after breakfast and coming home for supper with no explanation required about whatever transpired in the hours between. It was a different time, he recalls, where you trusted your neighbors and kids entertained themselves.

Every day, Jeffrey did just that, too. He filled his days with baseball, basketball, and football. He was naturally athletic, but his stature—small but mighty—always felt like a barrier. Despite this, Jeffrey kept at it.

Then, he found a sport where height did not matter one bit: racing cars. He took this newfound discovery and ran with it—or raced with it, rather. The adrenaline rush of high speeds thrilled him and kept him going back for more. He loved to go fast and felt drawn to anything that could get up and go.

Jeffrey spent the remainder of his childhood surrounded and molded by strong and encouraging women. Al Tasnady, the man who inspired him and grew to be a father figure, was the only exception.

DRIVE SLOW

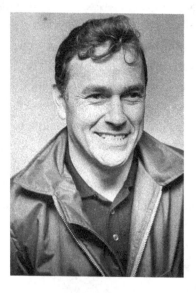

It is amazing how, on a day like any other, an important person can come into your life and change its course. In 1964

at age fourteen, Jeffrey met a famous stock car driver named Al Tasnady.

To fuel his need for speed and spend as little time as possible at home, Jeffrey started spending his time at the racetrack, admiring the greats from afar. Then, one day, things changed.

Jeffrey made his way to the parking lot after watching a race. He knew the big shots liked to hang out around their personal cars, shoot the shit, and have a beer or two after a race. Mustering up some courage, Jeffrey approached a parked 1960 Cadillac belonging to the one and only Al Tasnady. To this day, Jeffrey still remembers the license plate by heart: New Jersey FOY-800. The two got to talking, and simply put, Tasnady took a liking to Jeffrey and Jeffrey to Tas.

Tasnady was quite a name in the stock car space. He had a racing career full of accolades, including a spot in the Eastern Motorsport Press Association Hall of Fame. He was famous for his ability to control modified stock cars, like race cars with the body of a 1937 Plymouth (called "the Big Donkey") that had robust, modified engines and wide dirt track racing tires. Tasnady raced many cars over the years, but his favorite was the Big Donkey.

The so-called King of the Modifieds left his mark on and off the racetrack. Setting records and then breaking them repeatedly was Tasnady's forte. Though a ferocious competitor on the track, Tasnady had a soft side outside of racing and could charm a crowd like no other.

At the end of his astonishing driving career, Tasnady went on to become a renowned race director, continuing to leave his mark on the sport and young Jeffrey.

Although the pair had met, it was not until after Jeffrey's father died that the two became close. Tasnady sought Jeffrey out, intent on stepping in as a mentor and father figure. Tasnady had a way of connecting lessons learned on the track with those in life, communicating in a language that Jeffrey could easily understand.

"Drive slow, kid," Tasnady would say. He wanted Jeffrey to understand that life should never be taken for granted, and that as thrilling as it is to drive like the devil on an open highway, it is just as important to come off the pedal, slow down, and take it all in. Tasnady believed in appreciating all that you have and everything around you and never taking anything for granted.

Jeffrey absorbed this lesson, but he would not fully understand it until much later in life.

If it were not for Tasnady, Jeffrey is convinced he would never have become who is today. This talented man gave Jeffrey the ability to truly and deeply look at people—to listen and to understand them. Tasnady also passed down his people smarts, teaching young Jeffrey to be a master of charisma and confidence.

Jeffrey credits Tasnady with one of his most loved attributes, too, which is how to smile in a way that makes it so the other person cannot help but smile back.

Although he took in all sorts of life lessons on the track, traditional schooling felt lackluster and never held Jeffrey's attention. In the classroom, the cadence between the Fisher boys became that much more pronounced. Jan eventually dropped out of school in the tenth grade. Despite his troubles in school, Jan was a hard worker who was hell-bent on marching to the beat of his own drum. He went on to work in a glass factory and married at the age of sixteen when his girlfriend became pregnant.

Jeffrey made it through high school without investing too much time or energy into the idea of going to college. He was more interested in figuring out which races were worth running. All his life, he grew up going to the track and never saw himself on the path to higher education.

This all changed when he met Linda Knauer. Falling head over heels for her—his first love—Linda was going places and made it her mission to straighten Jeffrey out when it came to prioritizing his education. She had her sight set on Ivy League schools, and he started to see the possibilities of university life in a new light.

By his senior year of high school, Jeffrey realized that he enjoyed learning and was a promising student. Encouraged by Linda and her family, he started to entertain the thought of pursuing higher education but could not quite picture where or how.

Soon after, he met a neighbor named Bob Shofar, and the college idea came together. Bob attended Peirce Junior College in Philadelphia and enthusiastically sold Jeffrey on his alma mater. In an instant, Jeffrey made up his mind that he would enroll and never looked back. The first of his family to attend college, Jeffrey had yet to realize what a profound decision this would be for him.

COLLEGE

Walking into his interview at Peirce Junior College, though, Jeffrey was not prepared. Taking a page from Tasnady's playbook, he did what he knew best and sweet-talked his way through it. When he got his acceptance letter, the leading ladies in his life were simply ecstatic—the golden boy had hung the moon.

Peirce was a small college with all of two academic buildings and no dorms, which meant that Jeffrey shared a cramped house in New Jersey with his buddy and his wife. That did not last for more than one month. Jeffrey swiftly moved back home to Reading and commuted to school every day.

On his first day, Jeffrey had a rude awakening. Sitting in a room full of peers, the accounting professor walked in and immediately commanded silence from the chattering students. After a pause, he said, "Look to your left and then to your right. You will be one of two that graduates college."

Jeffrey had a single thought, *Oh, shit. I'm in trouble… big, big trouble.* Although his charms and intrinsic smarts had gotten him this far, Jeffrey realized he would have to do more than smile and charm his way through this one; he would have to work. And work hard to graduate. In that moment, he decided to be the one of two and successfully earn his associate's degree in marketing.

Day by day, lump by lump, Jeffrey found his feet at Peirce. By the end of his first year, he and his pal Jimmy Arnidis had gotten in the good graces of one of their favorite professors, Mr. Tony Falcone. What started as a chat around a class project evolved into a regular weekly meeting at The Sahara Bar on Fifteenth Street. Quite the dive, the Sahara was not much to look at, but it earned a soft spot in the boys' heart with stretched dollars going far enough to fuel late nights and animated discussions. Week after week, shared laughs and pints paid off, and the two best friends finished Falcone's class with As.

His close-knit cohort with Arnidis and Falcone taught Jeffrey that he loved learning through people. He had a knack for connecting and felt he got more out of rich conversations than he ever could from books. Subscribing to the social side of higher education, he sought to cultivate a more meaningful network among his peers.

Cue Greek life. To his dismay, pickings were slim when it came to choosing fraternities, and the options were simply not the right fit. Confident in who he was and what he wanted out of this affiliation, Jeffrey figured that if the right group didn't exist, he would simply have to make his own. Banding with his buddies Pete Gray, Ben Tursi, and Joe Tamney, the friends founded Theta Delta Epsilon and finally evened out the ratio of sororities and fraternities at Peirce. But he also had a secret: one of the driving factors behind Jeffrey being a founding member was that he did not want to go through hazing to pledge.

The process of bringing a new chapter to campus was much simpler back then. Jeffrey, with his friends in tow, marched down to the library—of all places—and got the approval from the head of the library, Dr. Jim McAuliffe. After that, they went to the director of activity, Fred Barfoot, for approval. The final step was to visit Dean Frank Pennypacker, and with all the members bought in, the new chapter was born. Theta Delta Epsilon was the newest chapter at Peirce and was chosen simply because the boys liked the name. Serving as social chair, Jeffrey was super involved with the chapter on and off campus. In between planning parties and having fun, Jeffrey also served as editor for Peirce's student-run newspaper, *The Peircetonian*. All told, these days were golden, and he loved every moment.

Upon graduating from Peirce with an associate of science degree in 1970, Jeffrey went on to attend Elizabethtown College in Elizabethtown, Pennsylvania, for two more years. Etown, as it is lovingly known, was a small Brethren college, and the only place that Jeffrey applied to that would accept his transfer credits from his program at Peirce. Jeffrey was motivated to get his bachelor's degree because he thought it would be an important factor in advancing his professional career after college. At this point, he also had no idea what he wanted to do, so he bought himself some time.

Admittedly, Jeffrey was not a fan of his new program for the entire first semester. The strict, dry campus was more work and less play than the bustling college life he had enjoyed at Peirce. Keeping his head down, Jeffrey resigned to slogging through in near misery until he met Jack Walton.

The yin to his yang, Walton was a science brainiac while Jeffrey was the marketing maven. The two played off each other's strengths and made their way through Etown as a team. Despite the tight reigns and Jeffrey's babyface, the duo never stopped seeking shenanigans and finding their fun together.

To add to his shenanigans while at Etown, Jeffrey was racing cars from eighteen to twenty-one years old with his best friend Robert "Griff" Griffith. With three years of driving fast and twenty races under their belts, the two were living their best lives. The thrill of racing lasted until Jeffrey was in a crash and hurt his back. It wasn't an extensive injury, but it made him reconsider and wonder, *Why am I even doing this? What's the point?* From there, Jeffrey's love for racing never died, but his drive to go fast dwindled, and he turned his focus elsewhere.

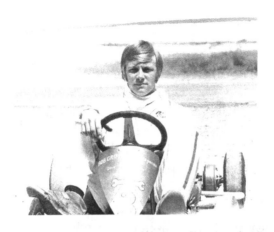

It was during this time that Jeffrey met Patti Scaringi in his second year at Etown. The two got along beautifully and their bond was based on friendship above all else. Eventually, Patti would become Jeffrey's first wife.

Jeffrey walked the stage and received his bachelor of science degree in marketing from Elizabethtown in 1972.

Ready for some practical experience to complement his college education, he dove into the workforce selling insurance at Metropolitan Life Insurance Company. This gig only lasted four months. Jeffrey hated how mundane each day was. After leaving the insurance business, Jeffrey's first love, Linda, proved to be a beneficial connection. Her father landed Jeffrey a job at Bachman Pretzels, which became his first introduction to the snack food industry.

Innately curious and now completely respecting the value of education, Jeffrey enrolled in St. Joseph's University Erivan K. Haub School of Business to secure his master of business administration. This third round was a different beast in the sense that he was committed to working full-time while earning his degree. But he was also not one to shy away from a challenge, and so he worked by day and attended classes at night to complete the program.

With an MBA in hand, Jeffrey entered the corporate world in 1980. He was energized, excited, and ready to take on the world.

Almost twenty years after entering the corporate world, Jeffrey missed the atmosphere of higher education. Inspired to go back, he applied and was accepted to the Wharton School of the University of Pennsylvania in Philadelphia, where he pursued an executive education degree and professional development certificate. This time, his studies consisted of more marketing, branding, leadership, and financial classes as opposed to a large focus on traditional business courses.

Nearly a decade later, Jeffrey was still itching to learn more. In 2008, Jeffrey received his professional qualification (PQ) from the Association to Advance Collegiate Schools of Business International Bridge Program. This was in cooperation with the Marshall School of Business of the University of Southern California; the Paul Merage School of Business of the University of California, Irvine; and Babson College. The PQ prepared senior business executives for academia and added to Jeffrey's extensive professional and academic résumé.

FAMILY

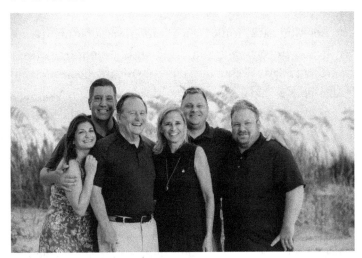

Jeffrey met his first wife Patti Scaringi in his fourth year at Etown, and the two were married on February 3, 1973. Conveniently, Tasnady retired on the same day, which meant Jeffrey's role model was able to be at his wedding to celebrate. Settling down in Reading, Pennsylvania, Jeffrey and Patti spent their time going to Maryland where Patti's family lived, racing, and traveling.

Ready for a family of their own but unable to conceive after two years, Jeffrey and Patti decided to adopt a baby in 1976. Their child was born on April 14, 1978, in Bogota, Colombia. Patti and Jeffrey's son Justin arrived in the United States three short weeks later, officially making the young couple a party of three.

As fate would have it, in January 1980, Patti found out that she was pregnant. Nine months later, Brandon was born on October 13, followed two years later by Trevor on January

13. Then, there were five in the family. Both boys were thought to be miracle babies, as Patti thought she was unable to get pregnant.

Looking back, while each addition was a bit unexpected in their own way, each son came with elation, overwhelm, and excitement. Eventually, Jeffrey built the house that the Fisher pack would grow up in on Museum Road in Mohnton, Pennsylvania, until the boys were ready to leave the nest.

Jeffrey's three boys were born within four years of each other. While this certainly made for some exciting times, each had their own distinct personality.

Justin is the oldest. Jeffrey and Patti adopted him in Colombia when he was just a few days old. Growing up, he was the quietest of the bunch. He was always patient and was a dedicated problem-solver. He could sit for hours trying to figure out how to put something together. He loved sports and played tennis during high school and college. Jeffrey and Patti loved how Justin would frustrate his opponent by always being able to return their shot, and the volleys could go on forever. Justin got his doctor of chiropractic medicine degree from the New York Chiropractic College. Despite Justin always being shy and quiet at home, he was quite the opposite around his peers. Everyone in his hometown of Charleston, South Carolina, seems to know and love Justin. Jeffrey and Alice teasingly called him the Mayor of Avondale. He now does CrossFit with the same patience and tenacity he had when he used to play tennis, and he is married to his lovely wife, Laura.

Up next is Brandon, the quintessential middle child. Brandon has always marched to the beat of his own drum. While the other boys loved less contact sports like baseball and tennis, Brandon decided that he was going to play football in high school. He always made a point to stand out from the pack. His adventurous outlook on life kept his parents on their toes and oftentimes pragmatic. Brandon insisted on snowboarding, but he gave up after his first fall. Then, he was going to start a band until Jeffrey sat him down to crunch numbers for the price of the tour bus that the band had their hearts set on. Brandon is also a people pleaser. He went to St. Joseph's University for food marketing, following in Jeffrey's footsteps. After graduating, Brandon kept his spontaneity alive and made an out-of-the-blue announcement that he was going to graduate school for politics at George Washington University. While politics seemed like a random choice, being the middle child had its advantages, and the important lessons had already been learned. Brandon was always having to negotiate between Justin and his younger brother, Trevor. This served him well with his work in politics. Brandon kept the family laughing—never failing to tease Jeffrey—and always doing his best impersonation of Chris Farley's *The Van Down by the River* sketch.

Trevor is the youngest. He loved playing baseball when he was younger and especially loved when Griff would come to his games. Trevor would always look for him decked out in his Dodgers gear in the stands. Griff was adamant about passing on his words of wisdom, such as "Break the second baseman's legs!" Trevor also loved WWE-style wrestling. His favorite wrestler was Hulk Hogan. Jeffrey would take him over to Griff's house to watch different events, and he would cry if the Hulk lost. Trevor went on to have a very successful tennis career during high school. He finished third in Pennsylvania in doubles and went on to play on scholarship in college. But he is still the typical "baby" of the family. In any conversation, everything always circles around to Trevor, and he knows it. Eventually, he cuts off questions about him.

When the boys were respectively twenty-one, nineteen, and seventeen, Patti and Jeffrey got divorced in 1999. The pair had simply drifted apart.

Fast forward to 2000, when Jeffrey met Alice Brommer. Having been pushed together at the racetrack by mutual friends, excitement has been the focal point of Jeffrey and Alice's story from the outset. One day, Alice offered to take Jeffrey on as a client through her travel agency.

Shooting his shot, Jeffrey quickly and subtly turned a work meeting into a lunch date. That was more than twenty years ago, and the couple has not stopped talking since. The Fishers were friends first and quickly became inseparable as their relationship blossomed. Marrying in May 2004, they kickstarted their life together in Reading, Pennsylvania, and ultimately settled down in North Carolina.

CAREER

Armed with extensive education in marketing and sales, Jeffrey was drawn to the snack foods industry, with a particular interest in meats. At the time, snack foods were an emerging fad that the country just could not get enough of. By the 1980s, snacking had become a leisure pastime that eventually emerged as an internationally recognized emblem of the American way of life, which set the stage for the snack food explosion.[1]

The early days of the snack food industry felt a bit like the Wild West. Requiring a certain type of scrappy and confident person to claw their way through a wide world of mixed nuts and snack packs, Jeffrey arrived hungry for success.

Jeffrey felt like he could make his mark in the snack foods bubble. Quickly finding his feet at Bachman Products, he was off to a new kind of race, clambering up the corporate ladder and soon joining the ranks of senior-level executives.

Over the course of his thirty-five-year career, Jeffrey held titles of regional and national sales manager, vice president of sales and marketing, vice president, executive vice president, and president. Staying on the East Coast, he enjoyed success in his beloved snack foods and meats industry from 1972 to 2011. He worked with industry giants like General Mills, Acme Foods, Knauss Snack Food, American Foods Group, and Godshall's Quality Meats.

Jeffrey's power play was maximizing success within his companies by developing effective strategies and refining talented personnel to achieve consistent prime performance. Simply put, he put people first. Among his colleagues, Jeffrey was recognized as a solid and conscientious leader who knew how to maximize and amplify the greatest asset for any entity: its people.

Jeffrey had the most success at Godshall's Quality Meats in Pennsylvania. The company was running smoothly, but the operations manager and eventual president, Ron Godshall, recognized that he did not have the sales experience necessary

---

[1]   https://www.wsj.com/articles/how-snacking-became-respectable-1377906874

to scale his company. Godshall's brought Jeffrey on as vice president of sales and marketing in 2010, and six short months later, he had increased overall sales by nearly thirty percent over the previous year. During his tenure, the sales of the company increased by $12 million.

CALLED TO TEACH

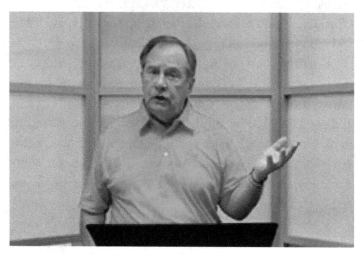

While at Acme Foods, one of Jeffrey's colleagues, Dale Falcinelli, was also an adjunct professor at Lafayette College and Lehigh University. They became good friends, and Dale's love for teaching was a constant point of conversation. Jeffrey's curiosity took over once again, and he began teaching college students.

Jeffrey felt as if he could add value to young minds and help the future generation be the best versions of themselves. He also loved to get up in front of people and just talk. And, boy, did he talk!

foothold in the corporate arena, he could not ignore his calling to teach.

Practicing patience and persistence, Jeffrey was finally presented with the opportunity to become a full-time professor at Elon.

NUMBERS GAME

Two hours later, Jeffrey was still unsure of what his decision would be. He loved the people at Godshall's but also loved teaching and his students at Elon.

What was the biggest obstacle in making a decision, though, was the pay.

Growing up in Reading, Pennsylvania, Jeffrey and his family didn't have much money. However, his mother and Grandmom always found a way to provide and make sure the boys had what they needed. This stuck with Jeffrey, and when he found himself more than comfortable financially, it was tough to accept a pay cut as consequence for pursuing his passion to teach.

The offer on the table from Elon was for less than half of his then salary as the vice president of sales and marketing at Godshall's.

Jeffrey and the dean, Dr. Bill Burpritt, went back and forth about raising the salary, but because he did not have a doctorate, there was not much that could be done. The numbers were firm, and there was no budge in the budget.

Jeffrey deliberated for well over a month. Every morning, he would wake up resolute, only to second guess his choice later in the day. It quickly became apparent that this was

While working, Jeffrey simultaneously served as an adjunct professor for sixteen years at three different schools. From 1997 to 2000, Jeffrey instructed marketing, sales, and business courses at Reading Area Community College in Pennsylvania. From there, he joined Lebanon Valley College, also in Pennsylvania, where he taught principles of marketing for eight semesters.

In 2007, Jeffrey's company, Knauss, moved to Martinsville, Virginia. Being on the border of Virginia and North Carolina, Jeffrey and Alice settled down on the North Carolina side in Whitsett.

During the transition, Jeffrey realized that he still loved to teach but did not know exactly how or where he would continue. Whitsett happened to be fifteen minutes from Elon University, so Jeffrey looked up open faculty positions at Elon for fun one day.

Voilà! There was an opening in the MBA program for a marketing professor. After meeting with the dean of the business department, Dr. John Burbridge, Jeffrey accepted an adjunct position.

Jeffrey taught at Elon University in North Carolina from 2007 to 2011. His teaching career blossomed as he served as a professor, as head of capstone programs, the MBA program, case studies, and executive education projects.

His students—his "kids" as he called them—were dynamic, capable, and teeming with promise. Elon's faculty, staff, and campus were more than ideal for Jeffrey. The school was everything that Jeffrey could have asked for in a teaching position.

Torn between two worlds, Jeffrey felt caught between business and education. Although he appreciated and respected his simply a numbers game—a matter of a five-figure versus a six-figure salary.

Growing up on the poorer side of an urban city, it was tough to consider giving up this six-figure salary he had worked so hard to bring home. The freedom of Jeffrey's executive salary gave him and his family the ability to travel often and spend time with relatives and loved ones far away. That was a lifestyle that was hard to beat.

By that point in life, Jeffrey was responsible for more than just himself, and he was worried that he would not be able to provide the same standard of living for himself or his dependents if he took the cut.

Looming large, the put-up-or-shut-up date was a week out and his decision was coming down to the wire. In the end, Jeffrey was never forced to make that choice—circumstances made it for him.

Seven days before the deadline, Jeffrey suffered a stroke.

STROKE

FATE WOULD HAVE IT

On Friday morning, September 2, 2011, Jeffrey woke up struggling to breathe.

Neither in pain nor feeling particularly panicked, he recalls simply not being able to take a deep breath. Mainly out of an abundance of caution, he and Alice loaded up in the car and went to the hospital in Greensboro, North Carolina. Quickly ushered back to a waiting room, the emergency room doctor ordered an EKG. The test results indicated there was a problem with Jeffrey's heart.

Being incredibly stubborn, Jeffrey could not accept the results. He argued with the doctor, starting what would go down as hours of debate between consultants and colleagues. Finally, they reached a consensus that a stent needed to be put in Jeffrey's heart.

The surgery was nonnegotiable, but he would have to wait until Monday. Not particularly thrilled with this lack of control over his care, Jeffrey pushed back. As fate would have it, there was a fluke opening for an operating room that day, so Alice and Jeffrey decided to have the surgery done then and there. Carpe diem—and get it over with.

When the doctor got the scope into Jeffrey's chest, he made it to his sternum before having to stop as there was a significant amount of plaque buildup. What happened next was a blur.

According to the doctor's account, the doctor broke up some of the plaque with the scope and caused it to race through Jeffrey's bloodstream up to his brain. Jeffrey suffered a massive stroke in the operating room.

Jeffrey had been partially awake for it all. Fading in and out, he remembers seeing his mother, who by that point, had been dead for decades. She kept repeating, "Go back! Go back! You're going to be fine."

"Fine" was generous.

The stroke occurred in the left frontal lobe of Jeffrey's brain, causing the entire right side of his body to become paralyzed. When he awoke, he opened his mouth to speak, but nothing came out. On top of the paralysis, his speech was impaired, and he was unable to read or write.

Jeffrey was terrified. He couldn't understand why Alice and his sons were constantly hovering. He kept trying to speak to them and communicate with them. Silence. He simply could not.

What was once his sword and shield, his brain and body were now a prison. Feelings and information came back to him in fragments without any rhyme or reason.

The initial diagnosis was aphasia, or brain damage, resulting in the loss or impairment of a person's ability to comprehend and communicate verbal language.

Due to the severity of his aphasia, the doctors opted to confer with Alice about what had happened in surgery, his diagnosis, next steps, and the long journey ahead. In an instant, the provider became the patient, and Alice was wholly responsible for Jeffrey's care and recovery.

The one thing you need to know about Alice is that she is a force. Small in size and slight in stature, Alice never shows externally the way she feels internally. Faced with the impossible odds and crushing possibility that the love of her life may never recover, she stayed calm, collected, and cool under the barrage of bad news and bleak prognoses from physician after physician.

Over the thirty-five endless days at the hospital, Alice never left Jeffrey's side. When she finally wheeled Jeffrey out of the automated doors, the real work began.

APHASIA

Aphasia is one of the most common and substantial conditions that can stem from a stroke. It is typically the result of brain damage to the left portion of the brain.

Aphasia can impair an individual's ability to speak, comprehend language, read, and write. It does not, however, impede or reflect intellect, which is part of what exacerbates the frustration and trauma hallmarked by this condition. Aphasia affects each individual in a unique way, and for many, whether they will recover is largely unknown following a diagnosis.[2]

In Jeffrey's case, it took him about two weeks to fully realize and understand what had happened to him as the doctors did not cite aphasia immediately. Once he received an official diagnosis, Jeffrey had no feelings of sadness or anger. He was strictly focused on what he had to do next to make it better. Despite doctors explaining everything about aphasia, it still did not sink in with Jeffrey that his life would never be the same. It wasn't until his time at the Sticht Center that he began to accept his new reality. At the center, he learned that the rest of his life would be a constant bettering and strengthening of himself.

Once reality had sunk in, Alice and Jeffrey worked together to make a plan and decide what would be best in terms of trying to recover. The first step, as they saw it, was to figure out to what extent the condition had affected Jeffrey. From there, they could move to rehabilitation, which would require finding the best doctors and therapists to help him.

The learning curve was steep, and the pair quickly found themselves taking a sharp left turn down a path with no map or guide.

---

[2]   Aphasia Voice

REHABILITATION PERIOD

Since the day of his stroke, Jeffrey has seen more than twenty doctors, therapists, and coaches. As Jeffrey put it, doctors are people, too. You have some good ones and some bad ones, and some you do or do not get along with.

Thus began the winding road from where Jeffrey's rehabilitation journey commenced and who he would spend his time with since that fateful September day.

Perhaps the most notable rehabilitation facility that Jeffrey attended was not a part of his life immediately following his stroke. Seven months into his recovery and two rehab facilities later, Alice reached out to Maura Silverman, speech and language pathologist and head of the Triangle Aphasia Project (TAP) in Cary, North Carolina.

TAP serves individuals with aphasia, their families, and the community through innovative life participation approaches that maximize communicative potential and reduce barriers to social re-engagement.[3]

In May 2012, Jeffrey began working with Maura. TAP's claim to fame was and remains the individualization of care, and Maura's approach proved to be just that in its unique, effective, and practical nature. Jeffrey was given real-life scenarios that were related to his topics of interest and applied them to his area of executive expertise. While this approach was more challenging, it was a turning point for Jeffrey's recovery because he was fully engaged. As he remembers it, Maura put Jeffrey through hell, and he absolutely loved it.

---

[3]   aphasiaproject.org

Other notable therapists who contributed to Jeffery's recovery were Katie Murphy, MS, CCC-SLP, and Rebecca Martin, both passionate specialists committed to helping people speak again.

Katie Murphy was leading a clinical trial at the Medical University of South Carolina for stroke victims. During their time together, Jeffrey improved most in discourse, conversational skills, public speaking, and self-confidence.

Rebecca Martin was a remote public speaking and communication coach based out of California. Jeffrey reached out to Rebecca in 2017 for speech and presentation coaching, and the two worked together for two years. Over this time, Jeffrey's confidence in speaking got a boost because he learned that others wanted to hear his story.

Despite his reservations, people could understand him as he spoke, and they were moved by his experience. His story helped bring to fruition some major themes in his life that had served not only as a foundation for who Jeffrey is today but also how he has remained so optimistic and on track in his journey to recovery.

To increase Jeffrey's chances of improvement, Alice found multiple unique types of rehab to help with particular issues. Jeffrey's stroke had affected the part of his brain that controlled his breathing. Jeffrey was having problems with the volume of his voice and getting enough oxygen to project. So, Alice thought singing and learning about the diaphragm would be a great way for him to tackle the issue. It certainly wasn't a pretty sound at first, but it was successful. Jeffrey even got to put on a show and sing his favorite Frank Sinatra song, "I've Got You Under My Skin."

Once settled in Charleston in 2017, Alice was walking their dog outside of their apartment complex and met a kind face. Alice struck up a conversation with Dr. Maysa Hannawi and, after many walks with their dogs, she found out that Maysa had recently graduated from the MUSC Physical Therapy school and had opened her own cash-based practice called In the Box PT.

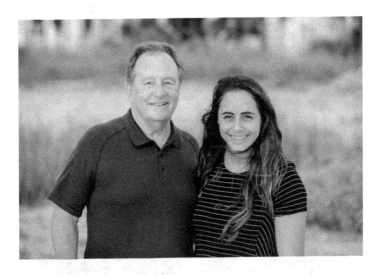

Alice knew Jeffrey had a lot of fight in him, so she continued to do everything she could to help him get better. One day, she finally recommended Jeffrey to see Maysa for physical therapy, especially since he hadn't been doing anything since they had moved. The first time that Maysa met Jeffrey, he was very eager. He was able to do tasks necessary for a limited but independent life, but he was still not able to do the things he wanted to truly enjoy an active life again. During their introduction, Maysa observed Jeffrey and discovered that he was only using the left side of his body and struggled greatly with talking. Once everyone was cleared with the apartment complex, Maysa and Jeffrey planned to meet in the on-site gym and begin.

This type of physical therapy was different than anything Jeffrey had done. This was a total mental and physical workout. In the past, many doctors had gotten him to do the bare minimum and that was it. Despite it being seven years poststroke, Maysa knew that they could do much more with what Jeffrey had. In starting this journey, Maysa was never worried or puzzled. She knew Jeffrey wanted to try everything and was never afraid of falling or failing. Maysa was the first person from a healthcare perspective to not treat him like he was broken.

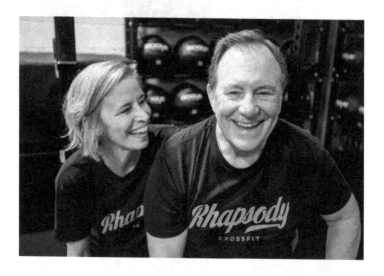

After continuing the good fight for six months, Maysa finally challenged Jeffrey to come with her to the place she always spoke about—Rhapsody Fitness. Starting out in one of Rhapsody's adaptive athlete events under the close eye of head coach and cofounder Alan Shaw, the one class eventually turned into one-on-one personal training sessions. Before long, the sessions turned into weekly classes. After some coaxing, Alice eventually joined in on the fitness fun, too.

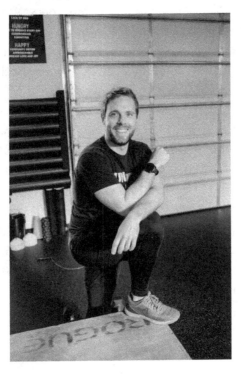

Having never touched a barbell before and not being able to jump, Alice and Jeffrey were definitely out of their comfort zones, but they leaned into the Rhapsody philosophy of adjusting and adapting to face the unknown. Despite the intense and seemingly impossible workouts, the community of Rhapsody athletes embraced Alice and Jeffrey and helped motivate them to continue. Today, everyone at Rhapsody knows their names. Everyone is friendly, welcoming, and supportive. It is truly a special place where judgement does not exist. Rhapsody has given Jeffrey and Alice a shared reason to continue to better themselves.

When Alice first started, she was scared to jump on a few plates. Now, she's climbing 15-foot ropes. When Jeffrey started, he couldn't get off the floor by himself. Now, he's doing burpees, walking lunges, and jumping rope. All of which have brought tears to the eyes of everyone on the sidelines in his life.

Looking back, Maysa's biggest accomplishment was getting Jeffrey to go into a CrossFit gym and showing him that he is truly capable. Accepting Maysa's challenge to join Rhapsody and work with Coach Alan, Jeffrey made an important choice about his life. He still makes a choice every single day to do all the hard things that get him closer to the life he wants through building strength, stamina, and mobility. Alan has the insight and drive to make everything work in a powerful and unique way. This drive, paired with Jeffrey's refusal to give up, has catapulted his recovery, which he continues to do every day.

PART II

KEY TAKEAWAYS

VANILLA MILKSHAKE |
PERSISTENCE AND
DETERMINATION

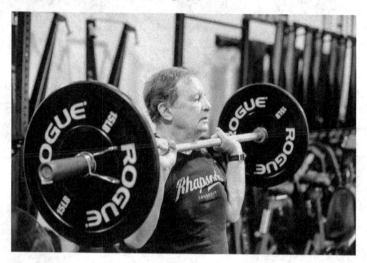

During his many hours of rehab with many practitioners, Jeffrey made a bet with Maura Silverman of the Triangle Aphasia Project. He told himself that once he was able to say, "vanilla milkshake," he would allow himself to order one. Simple, but not easy, this was a milestone that promised more than one sweet reward.

The terms of the bet were that Jeffrey had to order a vanilla milkshake himself, entirely unassisted, in order to claim his prize. If he tripped up or couldn't order the treat himself, then no milkshake. A tad cruel, the terms of this bet were finite. Multiple drive-through attempts and five long weeks later, Jeffrey triumphed and had the best damn vanilla milkshake of his life.

Persistence is defined as continuing a course of action firmly or obstinately in spite of difficulty or opposition. But to fully know and understand persistence past its simple dictionary definition, one must experience hardships. Through hardships and an abundance of trials and tribulations, it is only fair to say that those who push through truly and deeply know persistence.

Jeffrey understands and appreciates persistence on a deep level.

Before the stroke, Jeffrey displayed persistence in many ways. He was determined to be the best and help those around him be their best selves in the business world. Jeffrey would always do what was in the best interest of his company and coworkers, regardless of how difficult the circumstances were.

During their time together at Acme Foods, his friend and colleague Brian Flemming shared these values throughout their careers. The company had its ups and downs, but regardless of success or failure, Jeffrey always forged ahead with the same relentless determination to succeed and make progress. When it comes to determination and persistence, Jeffrey had written the book.

When his life was flipped upside down, persistence bubbled up with an entirely new set of demands and challenges—the stakes seemed higher than ever. The most amazing and telling example of his determination is how he has faced the effects of his stroke.

Many victims diagnosed with Jeffrey's degree of aphasia would have taken a different path to recovery—if not thrown their hands up and surrendered completely. When told by doctors that recovery was nothing short of hopeless,

Jeffrey and Alice simply refused to accept it. The couple started a decade-long journey that led them to the most respected doctors. The result of that persistence manifested in the remarkable improvement he has accomplished over the years.

Perhaps the most compelling reflection of Jeffrey's determination and persistence comes from speech writer and coach Rebecca Martin. Jeffrey sought out Rebecca's help in August 2017 for speech and presentation coaching. After a lengthy video call, Rebecca convinced herself and Jeffrey that they could reach his lofty goals. These seemingly impossible goals were pushed by Jeffrey's desire to speak the way he previously did before his stroke. He knew he would never be able to attain one hundred percent again, but anything above zero sounded amazing. So, with the odds stacked against him, Jeffrey pushed forward.

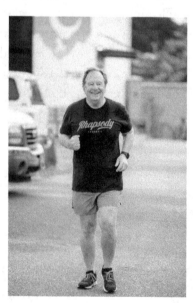

Jeffrey told Rebecca, "If you have the patience, I have the will to practice." He was driven by something greater than himself—his desire to help others who felt trapped and helpless just like he had for so many years. When his stroke first happened, Jeffrey's doctors emphasized that he was not going to be able to walk or speak again. It turned out to be exactly what he needed to hear to build his determination and prove them wrong.

Right then and there, he made the decision that he would speak and walk again no matter what it took. Doctors and diagnoses be damned.

Jeffrey has always identified as a persistent person and carried that characteristic with him poststroke. Although the definition of success may have changed, the man had not.

Having a stroke can be debilitating across the board, with many stroke survivors unable to return to their premorbid functions. However, in Jeffrey's case—progress continues to be gradual and improvements are ongoing. Jeffrey has never easily accepted the rejection of being told no.

Winston Churchill's famous quote, "Never, never, never give up," has been sitting on Jeffrey's desk as a magnet since 2012 and forever ingrained in his mind. From grinding his way through multiple colleges to become an educated man, working his way up in the corporate executive and teaching ladders to build his professional career, and now continuing to work hard at his recovery every single day, Jeffrey is no stranger to the importance and meaning of persistence and determination.

In his own words, "Staying persistent will always set you up for success as long as you are determined to do good things."

Some days, it may even reward you with a vanilla milkshake.

THE "P" STANDS FOR PRINCETON | CONFIDENCE

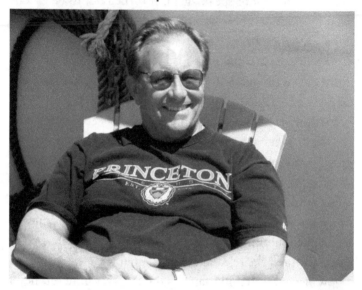

In 1996, Jeff Crowell sat down in the Marriott Hotel in Charlotte, North Carolina, for his interview with Knauss Foods. The interview was conducted by Jeffrey and his long-time colleague Brian Flemming. Naturally, Jeff was as nervous as a cat in a dog park. As he struggled to find a way to break the ice and rid himself of his anxiety, Jeff noticed the large gold "P" on the collar of Jeffrey's black mock turtleneck shirt.

Knowing Jeffrey was from Pennsylvania, Jeff asked if Jeffrey was a Pittsburgh Steelers fan. Jeffrey quickly corrected him and said, "The 'P' stands for Princeton."

Jeff was mortified, swallowed hard, and admitted his defeat. "Yep, there is certainly a difference." So much for getting off on the right foot.

Confidence can be a complicated topic—too much and you're cocky, but not enough and you may be seen as weak. Building confidence is also an intricate process that is often as unique to each of us as our fingerprints.

After his dad died, Jeffrey found himself under the wings of Al Tasnady. He instilled a confidence in Jeffrey like no one else. Tasnady's relentless racing style and constant hunger for success paid off and resulted in an impressive record, as well as a strong sense of self-confidence. Jeffrey, having spent many hours of his teenage years at the racetrack, modeled Tasnady, who showed him that this important trait is gained through experience—trial and error, rinse and repeat.

Before his stroke, Jeffrey saw himself on the top of the world when it came to sales and marketing in both of his roles as a business executive and a professor. He had reached a high point in his professional career in regard to measured success in the office and income he brought home. Jeffrey was comfortable and had surpassed the challenges of moving up the executive ladder no matter what obstacles he faced. As a professor, he was genuinely happy to share his knowledge of the professional world with the minds of tomorrow. Jeffrey had emerged at two different roads that presented him with two prestigious job opportunities. As a people person, he relied on his big personality to make a lot of things happen. For those around him, Jeffrey seemed to emit confidence.

He was professional, well-dressed, polished, and spoke with a silver tongue. Always driven and goal-oriented, he welcomed unique challenges and knocked them down like bowling pins after a clean strike.

Once, while taking a class at the Wharton School, he took a personality test to determine if he was more left-brained (analytical) or right-brained (creative/emotional). Jeffrey's results were split down the middle with a fifty percent attribution for each side. As he saw it, he was gifted with this perfect combination to help him succeed and was bred to be confident by divine design.

After his stroke, however, Jeffrey's confidence was stripped down to the bone in every way imaginable. For five years, he stayed at rock bottom. To him, confidence was no longer a tool available to him because he didn't know how to speak and was unsure if he ever would. His go-to reflex was gone.

Jeffrey felt lost trying to find his way back to his former self. He was unable to converse the same way he used to. Unable to connect the way he used to. It was like being in a crowded room and yelling, but no one was looking up. He began to understand just how dynamic and critical conversing and communicating were to him. All those years, he had taken his gift for granted.

Throughout this rough patch, he relied on Alice to speak for him. He was stricken with fear that he may never again be able to speak for himself.

After bouts of numerous speech therapists and facilities, Katie Murphy invited Jeffrey to join a speech and aphasia study being conducted at the Stroke Research and Education Center in the Medical University of South Carolina. The study was essentially to determine if concentrated speech therapy five days a week would be more beneficial to a participant instead of the traditional once or twice a week therapy protocol.

He started making progress, and with that progress came momentum. The momentum sparked something that started to look like confidence and was a turning point in his speech.

At first, the progress was slow, but then all at once, Jeffrey began to feel comfortable speaking in front of people because they all understood what was happening in his brain. He didn't have to work as hard to fill in gaps or rush through pauses—his audience was patient and knowing. Those with aphasia are not less intelligent, after all. They are wounded, and it is often that the general population does not understand this fact. In hindsight, Jeffery appreciates now that this was one of the reasons why regaining confidence had been so difficult.

In August 2017, Jeffrey and Alice reached out to Rebecca Martin for speech and presentation coaching. Building on his momentum from MUSC, rubber met the road in his speech recovery. Jeffrey wanted to empower others to take control of their own health and healing through speaking publicly about his journey with aphasia. In working with Rebecca, Jeffrey realized that people did want to hear his story and could gain something from it, so he started to tell it.

According to Rebecca, after each event and every speech, Jeffrey felt stronger. By the end of their time together, it was as if speaking in front of an audience came as naturally as it had before.

Jeffrey was then invited as the keynote speaker at the graduation of MUSC's occupational therapy department. In December 2019, Jeffrey stood in front of 175 bright-eyed graduate students and delivered an inspiring speech. By this point, he had regained eighty-five percent of his speech and was determined to make each word count. All told, the speech took him fifteen minutes to get through, but he did it with gusto and unbridled confidence.

What could have been the ultimate setback began a new era of inspiration and purpose. It was not until after he delivered his speech that he realized what he was meant to do, and that he had to lend his voice to those with aphasia.

Paul Squires, a professional associate to Jeffrey who became a personal friend, said, "He had a newfound confidence. He holds his head high again and is no longer concerned with what others think about him."

NO SMOKE AND MIRRORS | AUTHENTICITY

Authenticity is one of those qualities you must be all in on to pull off. Often requiring courage, it means that you show others your whole self, as opposed to select parts or polished aspects. A challenge in and of itself, when wielded well, authenticity creates space for genuine connection and deeper relationships.

Despite its high reward, authenticity does not come without risks—for many of us, fear of rejection tops that list.

Although he made a name for himself in a field stereotyped by people being anything but transparent and true, Jeffrey always identified as an authentic person. The marketing and sales space is known for being performative such that the sole goal could be achieved, which was to make the sale.

Jeffrey, however, learned early on that he could separate himself by defying the image of a typical marketer and salesperson. Instead of putting up smoke and mirrors, according to colleague and friend Paul Squires, Jeffrey was always genuine, straightforward, and honest, and he was a man of his word.

Jeffrey walked the walk on being authentic not only in sales and marketing but also in the classroom. He emphasized its importance and ethics to his students across the sales and marketing courses he taught. Staying the course paid off as he enjoyed long-term relationships with almost everyone he encountered across customers, colleagues, students, friends, and family.

Jeffrey had a way of making each individual think that they were the most important to him, and in that moment of time when he was with them, that was the truth. He would always take the time to listen and help wherever he could, whether it was with a business problem, a school inquiry, or a personal issue.

To him, authenticity and being direct went hand in hand. Jeffrey is known for not mincing words, even if the message is not easy to hear. Regardless, his bluntness proved to be helpful in the long run.

From his perspective, diplomacy was the key to beneficial authenticity, and the art of dealing with people in a sensitive and effective way was his key to success. Though he was always blunt, it is in the interest of others that this is tactfully paired with kindness and sincerity. As a devoted friend and mentor, Jeffrey found that his genuine nature had a calming effect on people, and he invited them to return it in kind.

Following his stroke, Jeffrey held onto his authentic self with even more fervor. Even though he also did not want to hear the truth he was told, he would make himself ask for it—insist on it, even—and absorb it. He developed a new appreciation for people being direct and authentic with him because everyone would try to sugarcoat his stroke, the rehab process, his quality of life, and his probability of returning to normalcy. Jeffrey demanded people to tell him how it really was no matter how hard it was to hear.

Jeffrey was forthcoming and honest about his situation with anyone who asked. He had aphasia, but he wanted nothing more than to tell his story to help others who were either suffering from the same condition or trying to support a loved one in a similar situation. At the start of his recovery process, though, being his authentic self was more difficult than he had expected because he was unable to express himself and communicate in the way he knew how.

On some days, he found it especially tempting to want to sweeten or skirt around the truth to protect either himself or the people he loved. On other days, it was a challenge to be authentic because he was getting to know parts of himself again that looked different after the stroke. He was the same, but he also was not. Having to dig into being authentic while becoming reacquainted with yourself is no easy task.

Early on, Jeffrey would try to do the things he had done before the stroke. A prime example was going back to work. It was entirely too soon for him to try going back, but he had to prove to himself that he could do it, even on a small scale. This led him to the realization that things were going to be different, and he started to be more comfortable with himself and where he was in his rehab journey. His goals shifted, yet his commitment to his core beliefs, his loyalty to his family and friends, and his resolve to be successful have never changed.

Another professional colleague and friend named Bill Fatica put it this way: "Jeffrey is the same person he was in

2002. It is important to never lose sight of your true self, no matter the situation."

Despite the hardship that he knew he would have to face for some time, Jeffrey did what he knew best—to do the next honest thing and show up as he was.

ADJUSTING THE SAILS | VULNERABILITY

A few months after his stroke, Jeffrey visited Paul Squires in his office. This was the first time he had seen his colleague since the stroke. Jeffrey squared his shoulders and walked through the door with a big smile on his face, but it was evident to Paul that he was extremely reluctant to speak due to the aphasia.

After a car accident had left him in a coma a few years prior, Paul felt like he could somewhat relate to Jeffrey. He invited Jeffrey out in hopes that he could offer a little guidance and direction. The next night, Paul and Jeffrey headed to the Hershey Hotel for dinner. It ended up being the most memorable encounter Paul had ever had with Jeffrey. Sharing a meal and traumatic experiences, Paul and Jeffrey's relationship transformed from one of professional associates to personal friends because of the openness, and above all, vulnerability they shared.

For Jeffrey, his unbridled drive came hand in hand with a fierce sense of independence. He believed he could do anything by himself, whatever "it" was, and never wanted to ask for assistance. Jeffrey's calm, cool, and controlled approach to thoughts, words, and ultimately actions is what got him to where he wanted to be in all parts of his life.

However, as these things go, this all changed for him. Jeffrey identifies with experiencing two searing types of vulnerability following his stroke. First, he was susceptible to physical and emotional harm. Second, he was in need of special care, support, and protection due to the aphasia and the lasting effects of his stroke.

For Jeffrey, this new reality of needing to ask for help so often was awful. It went against everything he had been taught and prided himself on. It was a muscle he had simply never learned to flex.

When faced with a seemingly insurmountable challenge, Jeffery did the last thing that came to mind—he laughed about it. Through humor, he was able to make light of a dark situation and found a way to be vulnerable with those around him. It was difficult at first, but as time went on, he found it easier to make light of the snags and eventually found himself feeling a bit lighter in heart.

Jeffrey feels he came into his own by talking about his fears and insecurities. When he first reached out to Rebecca Martin for speech and presentation coaching, she noted that he was completely vulnerable, and that this vulnerability was uncharted territory for such a guarded businessperson.

Jeffrey continued to come back to the question, "Do you think I can do it?" He was fiercely committed to telling his story, but he was unsure as to whether it was feasible.

Embracing this vulnerability and learning how to use it to his advantage, Jeffrey did not simply accept his circumstances. He took a life altering experience that could have filled him with anger for the rest of his life and instead leaned into the vulnerability to fuel a new life with a new set of passions. By finding the courage to be vulnerable, Jeffrey learned to hold a space for others to truly see him, connect with him, and support him. It's necessary to make yourself vulnerable to grow.

PARTNERSHIP PART I | FRIENDS

A friend is a gift you unknowingly give to yourself. These are the family you choose—the people in your life with whom you share your highest highs and lowest lows. When you attract those good eggs, they will challenge you to be better and carry you when you need it.

For most of us, friendship is essential. It is the sweet stuff that makes life worth living. But we may not truly appreciate just how important this chosen family is until the chips are down.

Jeffrey's list of good friends is pages upon pages long with countless stories and shenanigans paired with each person. Spanning college years to present day, every individual on that list has played a part in his life. Oftentimes, Jeffery suspects his inner circle knows him better than he knows himself.

To put this into perspective and dive deeper into who he is as a person, a friend, a businessperson, a teacher, a mentor, and a survivor, some of his dearest friends, pre- and poststroke, weighed in on the values and characteristics that Jeffrey embodies. While the list is lengthy, there is a common thread among each name—a defined pattern of honesty, determination, and intelligence. Other characteristics prevalent in the group include integrity, humility, self-confidence, moral centeredness, loyalty, conscientiousness, competence, engaging charm, authenticity, passion, dynamism, and sincerity.

In short, Jeffrey holds this group in the highest regard, and after understanding how they have weaved themselves into his life and walked alongside him in his journey, it is clear why. Jeffrey admits that he embodies all these qualities, thanks to his friends' examples.

Despite this collection of wonderful humans, three in particular had a profound effect on Jeffrey: Bob "Griff" Griffith, Howard Rissmiller, and Rick Weisser.

GRIFF

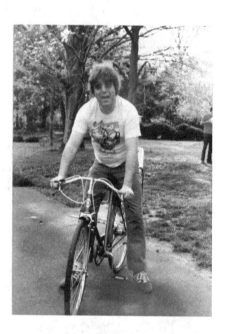

Jeffrey met Griff when they were just kids on the playground at Eleventh and Pike in Reading, Pennsylvania, in their early teen years. Griff was a wild man who never failed to find the fun and adventure that surrounded him. As the two grew up, this dynamic duo moved their party from the playground to the racetrack, which eventually led to their first big purchase: a go-kart.

Growing up, the pair did not go a single day without talking. Griff kept Jeffrey on his toes and taught him how to let go, be present, and just have fun. Frick and Frack were always laughing at or with each other. Griff was an indispensable friend. He took everything to the max and made the small things larger than life. Especially his love for the LA Dodgers. As an adult, he was quite the dedicated fan. Unfortunately, there was no way to get the Dodgers' games on television in Reading, Pennsylvania, in the 1980s, and Griff became known for the monstrous satellite dishes installed on the roof of his suburban row home. Although it looked as if he had set up a station to talk to astronauts in space, he simply watched his Dodgers—but in a big way.

HOWARD

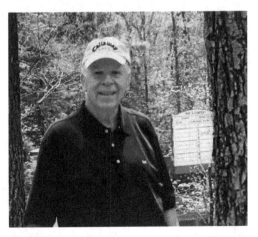

Howard and Jeffrey got to know each other through mutual friends in the food industry. As a baby in the marketing and sales world at thirty-two-years-young, Jeffrey expected to be surrounded by older and wiser colleagues. Ten years his senior, Howard took a shine to Jeffrey and showed him the ropes.

It took some time, but over the years Howard and Jeffrey formed a bond that was rooted in mutual respect and humor. Jeffrey attributes Howard with teaching him how to embrace being authentic in the boardroom and weaponizing his smile. Howard had a way of putting and keeping things in perspective, which grounded and comforted everyone around him.

He was so grounded and comfortable that Howard was entrusted with giving all three of Jeffrey's boys "the talk" as they went to college. He took great care to impart words of wisdom. Fondly, each boy was dropped off by Jeffrey at Howard's house, and they would go off on a walk and return with nuggets of advice that would carry them through life.

RICK

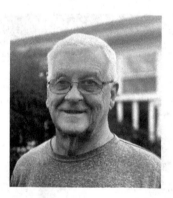

Rick and Jeffrey met in junior high school in 1962 in Reading, Pennsylvania. As young teens, they would race model cars, play multiple sports, and venture to stock car races together. Upon graduation, Jeffrey went on to Pierce Junior College, and Rick went to work straightaway in banking. On holidays and summer breaks, the two continued going to races together and they even got into racing go-karts; Jeffrey drove, and Rick strategized.

As time marched on, the pair grew up and drifted apart. In the early 1970s, they both got married and started living separate lives. From that point up until Jeffrey's stroke, there was a significant lull in their relationship that had been stripped down to limited contact and time together.

After the stroke, Jeffrey and Alice moved back to Reading, Pennsylvania. Rick and Jeffrey reconnected with his old friend over good food and warm conversation. The greatest lesson Rick taught Jeffery was consistency. Though Jeffrey understood that consistency pays off on many fronts, both personal and professional, it wasn't until his stroke and subsequent rehab journey that he truly appreciated the life lesson his friend had taught him.

Rick is steady and stable. Knowing that he's always there has given Jeffrey a sense of safety and security.

These friends, or chosen family, gave Jeffrey stories, shared experiences, challenges, empathy, and support when he needed it the most. Though these three friends each helped shape Jeffrey into who he is today, the three friendships were each very distinct. Simply put, they went through different seasons of life together.

Griff and Jeffrey were coming of age while racing go-karts and playing on the playground, while Howard helped Jeffrey move his things after his divorce with his first wife. Rick was there for all of it and still is to this day.

Blending a chosen family with real family, Jeffrey's sons all had relationships with these lifelong friends, too, and the boys loved them.

Unfortunately, as they say, only the good die young. Jeffrey was with Howard the day that he died. They sat in the front room of Howard's home together and spoke about life and death. Howard passed away after a battle with Non-Hodgkin's lymphoma in 2012 at the age of seventy-one. Griff died of a heart attack when he was just fifty years old in 1997. Whether his heart attack was due to a blocked artery or his beloved LA Dodgers losing is still up for debate. While his death was unexpected, it was the easier of the two to deal with because Jeffrey's time with Griff had a longer history.

Rick is still loving life and lives in Reading, Pennsylvania. He and Jeffrey talk often and share old stories over meals every time Jeffrey is in town.

If anything can be learned through solid friendships, numerous life lessons, and an abundance of warming memories, it's that partnerships are needed in all facets of our lives—none of us make it through alone. It is important to know that friends come and go, but there are a precious few you should cling to. Always work hard to overcome distance and lifestyle because you never know when you will need that circle of people to weave invisible nets of love that lift you up when you are weak and celebrate you when you are strong.

PARTNERSHIP PART II | ALICE

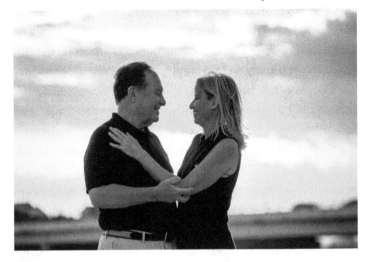

Friends are the family you choose, and then there is your partner—that best of friends you choose to live life with. Enter Alice.

From the start, Alice and Jeffrey's relationship revolved around love, excitement, and fun. Seven years after kick starting their life together, the true test of the "in sickness and in health" part of the wedding vows came into the equation with Jeffrey's stroke.

Before the stroke, Alice describes Jeffrey as caring, loving, considerate, and playful. He was never overly emotional, but he always treated Alice like his best friend, the most important person in the world, and his teammate. It never took much to bring out Jeffrey's smile—he was happiest at home or at the beach. Jeffrey never really sweated the small stuff, and he rarely even noticed it.

One Christmas, Alice had put up and decorated a spectacular tree for the season, but Jeffrey's reaction was to tell her that it was crooked. Despite sometimes missing little things here and there, Alice and Jeffrey were rock solid, and still to this day, they have never had a fight. Maybe a disagreement, but the two usually end up laughing by the end.

People often cannot stop asking why when something inexplicably terrible and unexpected happens to a loved one.

When Jeffrey came out of the operating room, and the doctors explained to Alice what had happened, she was initially terrified. Terrified that he wouldn't wake up, that she was going to make the wrong decision in the critical hours of his stroke, and that Jeffrey was going to react badly to what was promising to be a serious challenge for them both.

Then came the anger. Alice was angry with herself for agreeing to the procedure, despite her gut feeling that it was not necessary and was a bad idea. She was angry that the stroke happened at all.

Then came the despair. The feeling of loneliness and solitude crept in when Alice realized she did not have family in the area for support and had to make difficult and critical decisions on her own. Alice also felt an enormous amount of frustration and exhaustion. Getting Jeffrey into one of the best rehab facilities in the country was no small feat, and despite her strong spirit, Alice was tired.

Once out of the first hospital and into the rehabilitation process, Alice's emotions shifted. Frustration remained prevalent, but that was because there was no tried-and-true system in place to navigate the rehab necessary for stroke patients. Alice found herself more determined than ever to find any and every way possible, both conventional and nonconventional, to help Jeffrey get better.

Being a caregiver means mastering patience. It involves a lot of pressing and letting off the gas pedal. Then, somewhere along the way, one long day after another, an unexpected feeling started to seep in: elation. When Jeffrey had any kind of success, she was elated. And then there was pride. She was proud of Jeffrey for never saying no, always giving it his all, and showing his willingness to move onto something new.

Along with all of this, being a caregiver also means you may find yourself alone at times in your new leadership role and driver of another's care plan. Once Jeffrey had recovered enough to be moved into a regular room and out of the ICU, Jeffrey and Alice had visitors. Alice's sister-in-law and niece stopped in on their way home from a soccer game to see how things were going. They were the closest relatives Alice and Jeffrey had nearby. Even then, they were over two hours away. It was at that moment that the enormity of the situation hit Alice. She was overjoyed to see her family, but it was also the moment when she realized that she and Jeffrey were alone in this journey. Without question, Alice knew that Jeffrey would need a lot of rehab and that he would be determined to recover as much mobility and speech as possible. After one meltdown at the hospital, Alice took a deep breath and started researching and asking questions.

Oftentimes your partner's emotions are reflected and projected by the other. In Alice and Jeffrey's story, this is most definitely the case.

What does Alice believe makes for a successful partnership? To Alice, partnership means loving each other no matter what happens, always doing the small and large things for each other, and always supporting each other's decisions, opinions, and choices. Understanding that an opinion is just that—an opinion—and that by definition, it cannot be right or wrong. Partnership is recognizing something as being important to both people if it starts out as being important to one. Collaborative decision-making and thinking about the consequences for both parties is partnership.

Perhaps most importantly, Alice feels that you have to rely on each other to do your own part to make the partnership strong, worthwhile, and successful.

Jeffrey has always been Alice's best friend, and he was her knight in shining armor when she was in a very dark place. However strong initially, their partnership only grew after the stroke. Beforehand, they were both driven and independent people, who enjoyed sharing experiences but remained independently happy.

However, after the stroke, the two were forced to reassess their priorities, and at the end of the day, they realized that they were the most important thing to each other. From swimming across an ocean to moving a mountain, either would do anything for the other. This next chapter forced the pair to reevaluate how they relied on each other. Alice and Jeffrey's roles in their partnership have changed, but they have each adapted to their new roles and support each other always.

In many interviews, Alice was credited for being the driving force behind Jeffrey pushing himself to get to where he is now. Learning early on that traditional rehab was not going to help Jeffrey get to where he wanted to go, Alice was always looking beyond the obvious to find ways for him to get better.

She admits that she can be a real pain in the ass but knows the result will be worth it. While Alice has always been there to support and love Jeffrey and help him do his exercises or homework, he has been the true engine behind his own rehab. The success, ultimately, has been the collective effort of an unbreakable, unwavering partnership.

PART III

WHERE JEFFREY IS TODAY
AND WHAT'S NEXT

LIVING HIS BEST LIFE

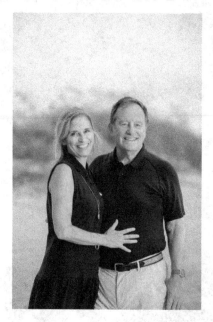

At first, Jeffrey's biggest motivation to continue the grueling process of rehabilitation was the desire to get back to who he was before the stroke and regain his hold on his executive and teaching careers. At the Aphasia Center, Jeffrey was solely there to focus on regaining the ability to lead the life he had had before the stroke.

Eventually, Jeffrey managed to get back in the classroom. He was invited to speak at Thomas Jefferson University and educate his audience on what aphasia was and what it meant to live with it. Six months later, he was asked to do a second part of the series via Skype before video conferencing became the thing to do. In this, Jeffrey was able to truly share what his daily life with aphasia was like by showing his home and routine. For the remainder of that year, Jeffrey continued his supportive. It is truly a special place where judgement does not exist. Rhapsody has given Jeffrey and Alice a shared reason to continue to better themselves.

When Alice first started, she was scared to jump on a few plates. Now, she's climbing 15-foot ropes. When Jeffrey started, he couldn't get off the floor by himself. Now, he's doing burpees, walking lunges, and jumping rope. All of which have brought tears to the eyes of everyone on the sidelines in his life.

Looking back, Maysa's biggest accomplishment was getting Jeffrey to go into a CrossFit gym and showing him that he is truly capable. Accepting Maysa's challenge to join Rhapsody and work with Coach Alan, Jeffrey made an important choice about his life. He still makes a choice every single day to do all the hard things that get him closer to the life he wants through building strength, stamina, and mobility. Alan has the insight and drive to make everything work in a powerful and unique way. This drive, paired with Jeffrey's refusal to give up, has catapulted his recovery, which he continues to do every day.

head coach and cofounder Alan Shaw, the one class eventually turned into one-on-one personal training sessions. Before long, the sessions turned into weekly classes. After some coaxing, Alice eventually joined in on the fitness fun, too.

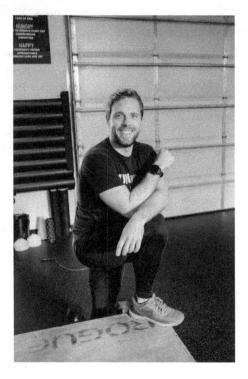

Having never touched a barbell before and not being able to jump, Alice and Jeffrey were definitely out of their comfort zones, but they leaned into the Rhapsody philosophy of adjusting and adapting to face the unknown. Despite the intense and seemingly impossible workouts, the community of Rhapsody athletes embraced Alice and Jeffrey and helped motivate them to continue. Today, everyone at Rhapsody knows their names. Everyone is friendly, welcoming, and with talking. Once everyone was cleared with the apartment complex, Maysa and Jeffrey planned to meet in the on-site gym and begin.

This type of physical therapy was different than anything Jeffrey had done. This was a total mental and physical work-out. In the past, many doctors had gotten him to do the bare minimum and that was it. Despite it being seven years poststroke, Maysa knew that they could do much more with what Jeffrey had. In starting this journey, Maysa was never worried or puzzled. She knew Jeffrey wanted to try everything and was never afraid of falling or failing. Maysa was the first person from a healthcare perspective to not treat him like he was broken.

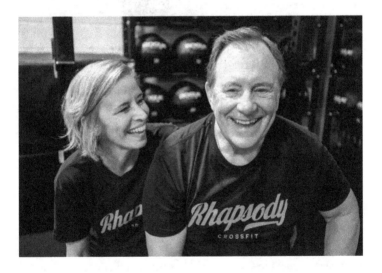

After continuing the good fight for six months, Maysa finally challenged Jeffrey to come with her to the place she always spoke about—Rhapsody Fitness. Starting out in one of Rhapsody's adaptive athlete events under the close eye of

Once settled in Charleston in 2017, Alice was walking their dog outside of their apartment complex and met a kind face. Alice struck up a conversation with Dr. Maysa Hannawi and, after many walks with their dogs, she found out that Maysa had recently graduated from the MUSC Physical Therapy school and had opened her own cash-based practice called In the Box PT.

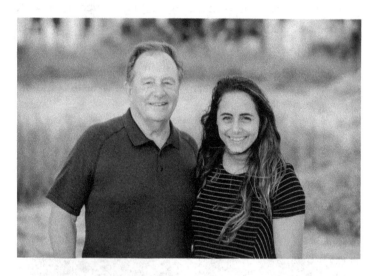

Alice knew Jeffrey had a lot of fight in him, so she continued to do everything she could to help him get better. One day, she finally recommended Jeffrey to see Maysa for physical therapy, especially since he hadn't been doing anything since they had moved. The first time that Maysa met Jeffrey, he was very eager. He was able to do tasks necessary for a limited but independent life, but he was still not able to do the things he wanted to truly enjoy an active life again. During their introduction, Maysa observed Jeffrey and discovered that he was only using the left side of his body and struggled greatly

Aphasia can impair an individual's ability to speak, comprehend language, read, and write. It does not, however, impede or reflect intellect, which is part of what exacerbates the frustration and trauma hallmarked by this condition. Aphasia affects each individual in a unique way, and for many, whether they will recover is largely unknown following a diagnosis.[2]

In Jeffrey's case, it took him about two weeks to fully realize and understand what had happened to him as the doctors did not cite aphasia immediately. Once he received an official diagnosis, Jeffrey had no feelings of sadness or anger. He was strictly focused on what he had to do next to make it better. Despite doctors explaining everything about aphasia, it still did not sink in with Jeffrey that his life would never be the same. It wasn't until his time at the Sticht Center that he began to accept his new reality. At the center, he learned that the rest of his life would be a constant bettering and strengthening of himself.

Once reality had sunk in, Alice and Jeffrey worked together to make a plan and decide what would be best in terms of trying to recover. The first step, as they saw it, was to figure out to what extent the condition had affected Jeffrey. From there, they could move to rehabilitation, which would require finding the best doctors and therapists to help him.

The learning curve was steep, and the pair quickly found themselves taking a sharp left turn down a path with no map or guide.

---

[2] Aphasia Voice

Jeffrey was terrified. He couldn't understand why Alice and his sons were constantly hovering. He kept trying to speak to them and communicate with them. Silence. He simply could not.

What was once his sword and shield, his brain and body were now a prison. Feelings and information came back to him in fragments without any rhyme or reason.

The initial diagnosis was aphasia, or brain damage, resulting in the loss or impairment of a person's ability to comprehend and communicate verbal language.

Due to the severity of his aphasia, the doctors opted to confer with Alice about what had happened in surgery, his diagnosis, next steps, and the long journey ahead. In an instant, the provider became the patient, and Alice was wholly responsible for Jeffrey's care and recovery.

The one thing you need to know about Alice is that she is a force. Small in size and slight in stature, Alice never shows externally the way she feels internally. Faced with the impossible odds and crushing possibility that the love of her life may never recover, she stayed calm, collected, and cool under the barrage of bad news and bleak prognoses from physician after physician.

Over the thirty-five endless days at the hospital, Alice never left Jeffrey's side. When she finally wheeled Jeffrey out of the automated doors, the real work began.

APHASIA

Aphasia is one of the most common and substantial conditions that can stem from a stroke. It is typically the result of brain damage to the left portion of the brain.

series at Thomas Jefferson, updated his audience on how he was doing, and what had or had not changed with him, since people did not know what aphasia was—he was both an educator and a living case study.

From the time he woke up unable to speak in the hospital to now, Jeffrey has taught six classes. When he was getting back into the swing of things, he couldn't talk very well, and it proved to be slow and difficult. The different audiences' reactions were always fascinating to him. They knew that he couldn't speak fluidly, but they also knew that he had it in him to talk. He wasn't able to verbalize or pronounce anything proficiently at the start, so the audience stayed engaged and helped him out by asking a lot of questions. Teaching these six classes is the only thing that Jeffrey has been able to get back to from his "old life."

In 2016, Jeffrey attended an international marketing class at Villanova University in Philadelphia taught by Dr. Charles Taylor. It quickly became apparent to Jeffrey that there was no way he could get back to teaching. So, he shifted his focus. The following year, Jeffrey came up with Aphasia Voice, an advocacy and education initiative. His idea quickly formulated and became real.

Aphasia Voice (www.aphasiavoice.com) is an education and advocacy initiative that discusses aphasia and Jeffrey's personal experiences. The venture came about because Jeffrey thought it would be interesting and beneficial to educate anyone interested (therapists, doctors, students, etc.) on all aspects of the condition. Since its inception in 2017, Jeffrey has completed about twenty presentations for or through Aphasia Voice to tell his story and educate the audience.

Jeffrey is still that same driven person that he always was, except now his drive is for a much different reason. While before he was focused on success in business and teaching, Jeffrey is now focused on his need to get better in body and in speech. His stroke happened ten years ago, but he has never given up trying to recover in every way possible.

If Jeffrey were to take the same personality test that he did at the Wharton School, the results would be much different. Due to the damaged area in the left side of his brain, the right (creative/emotional) side has taken over. Jeffrey is much lighter and easily brought to laughter. He will do things to get anyone and everyone to smile and laugh at his antics—so much so that he now plays the air guitar and dances. He is also much more emotionally in tune and demonstrative with his feelings. Jeffrey no longer worries about previous stressors from his prestroke life. The only thing he worries about is his rehabilitation, and the numbers game is no more—it is a quandary that resolved itself.

These days, Jeffrey's happiness is ever-present and overflowing. He is simply happy when he wakes up in the morning. Before his stroke, he still woke up happy, but it was in a different way and for different reasons. Today, when his happiness hits a wall, he takes a nap and wakes up even happier. For five years following his stroke, Jeffrey had hit a bit of a slump. He wanted desperately to get involved with things that once made him who he used to be, but he knew these things were impossible. Eventually, Jeffrey came to terms with his reality. In regard to work life, he no longer does anything related to his old executive profile.

Charleston offers an abundance of activities and opportunities to try new things. Jeffrey fills his free time with workouts at Rhapsody Fitness, physical therapy sessions with Dr. Maysa Hannawi, classes two days a week at the College of Charleston, meetings with the Aphasia Support Group at MUSC, collaborating with Aphasia Recovery Connection on Facebook, horseback riding at Rein and Shine once a week, refining his public speaking with Dr. Grace Privette-Farren, spending time with his sons every weekend, and of course, hanging out with Alice and their two dogs, Hannah and Mia. It is safe to say that his dance card is full.

Jeffrey's favorite part about poststroke life is that he can sit when he needs to sit, but he stays active. Simply put, he is always doing something unless he is sleeping. Jeffrey does not let any time go to waste.

Jeffrey and Alice have hopes of traveling to Italy and Switzerland for the first time and make it back to Maine someday. Jeffrey looks forward to continuing to learn from his sons and hopes that one day, he can convince them to come join Rhapsody Fitness.

When it comes to life goals, Jeffrey has set the bar high. Gaining a sense of purpose and life to be healthy and happy over ninety is at the top of his list. Jeffrey wants to hold onto Dr. Maysa Hannawi and Rhapsody coach and cofounder Alan Shaw until he is at least seventy-five as they are both special people to him.

On top of all these exciting developments, the year 2021 brought Jeffrey's story to the big screen with the help of Alan and Trinity from Rhapsody Fitness and David and Noah from Matchlight Production Company. For Alice and Jeffrey both, it was an honor to be featured with their favorite gym. Going forward, Jeffrey wants to use the video and his memoir, both lovingly titled *Never Give Up*, to help educate the world about aphasia. He also hopes to use Aphasia Voice for outreach and to get his foot in the door for more speaking engagements.

Most importantly, Jeffrey will continue to endlessly love and trust Alice, Justin, Brandon, Trevor, Lauren, Hannah, Mia, and whoever else comes into his life. After all, love and trust serve as reminders that you are never in it alone.

APPENDIX

REHABILITATION FACILITIES, PROVIDERS, AND PROGRAMS:

- Moses Cone Hospital: September 2011
- Sticht Center at Winston Salem Hospital: September 2011
- Alamance Regional Hospital- Rehabilitate: October–November 2011
- Moses Cone Hospital–Rehabilitate: January–February 2012
- Dr. Jeffrey Marrongelle: March 2012–present
- Maura Silverman MS, CCC-SLP and the Triangle Aphasia Network: May 2012–April 2013
- Professor Scott Nice, University of North Carolina, Wilmington: August 2013–January 2014
- Kerri Connell, MA, CCC-SLP: September 2013–December 2013
- Dr. Gigi McDonald: September 2013–August 2014

- The Aphasia Center: April–June 2014
- Joan Schwanger, MS, CCC-SLP: February 2015–September 2016
- Lingraphica: March 2015–February 2017
- Reading Hospital, Dr. Claire Flaherty: May 2015–February 2017
- Susan Lynch, MA, CCC-SLP at The Magee Center: September 2015–February 2017
- Dr. Ronald Herb: September 2015–present
- Dr. Roy Hamilton, University of Pennsylvania: October 2015
- David Bossler, SCORE: October 2015–February 2017
- Mary Detweiler at The Moss Center: February 2016–February 2017
- Karen Cohen, MA, CCC-SLP: February 2016–February 2017
- Paula Sobel, MA, CCC-SLP: February 2016–February 2017
- Sharon Mast, May 2016–February 2017
- Susanne A. LeCoure: June 2016–December 2016
- Dr. David Ermak: February 2017
- Katie Murphy, MS, CCC-SLP: May 2017–present
- Rebecca Martin: August 2017–December 2019
- Rein and Shine: September 2017–February 2019
- Dr. Maysa Hannawi: October 2018–present
- Kikki Thayer, MS, CCC-SLP: January 2019–November 2019
- Rhapsody Fitness: June 2019–present

"THE LAST LECTURE" GIVEN AT MUSC'S SCHOOL OF OCCUPATION COMMENCEMENT

Three years ago, I came to this place, MUSC. Being here changed my life. I want you to know that you will have the opportunity to change people's lives in the future.

They asked me if I wanted to participate in the Occupational Therapy Stroke Boot Camp. I'll do it!

You know, you students were so special. So special. I loved your cheerfulness. You were exuding. You did everything from teaching me how to fix a shirt to how to tie my shoes. I actually thought you were the most dedicated people I had ever met in my life. You treated me with care, and that is how I liked it.

I am honored to be speaking to you today because I am one of two million people with aphasia who could not talk. I got better because of people like you.

Hi, my name is Jeffrey Fisher. I am from Charleston, South Carolina.

I have aphasia. I have worked for eight years to be able to talk to you like I'm doing today. And today I will tell you a little bit about my story. What has happened along the way. What I have done to recover. And the lessons I learned along the way.

Before I went to the hospital, I was doing well financially. I was a vice president of sales and marketing for Godshall's Quality Meats Company. I was an adjunct professor of marketing at Elon University.

That Friday before Labor Day in 2011, I couldn't catch my breath. So, I went to Moses Cone Hospital in Greensboro, North Carolina. Unfortunately, my doctor was out that day. This was a new doctor. And I did not know him.

So, I was hooked up to the EKG. When we were finished, he said, "I have some bad news for you. It's your heart." I said, "My heart? You have got to be kidding me. I don't have a heart problem!"

He said he wanted to put a stent in my heart. I said, "I don't believe it, I just don't believe it."

It got heated—really heated. We went back and forth for thirty or forty-five minutes. And then, I decided to go to the hospital and sign the papers. I was feeling very negative about the surgery.

When I woke up, the whole right side of my body was paralyzed. And they never put the stent in my heart. Proving that I did NOT have a heart problem to begin with. I tried to speak, and nothing came out. Uh oh, we have a problem.

Six days later, my wife and son Bo took me to the Aphasia Center in Winston Salem, North Carolina. This was the beginning of a long, long journey. I just kept telling myself, *I'm going to get better. I'm going to get better. I'm going to get better.*

I was at the Sticht Center for twenty-one days. After twenty-one days, the doctors realized what a BIG problem I had. But because of my insurance, I had to leave.

At first, I was stubborn. I wanted to get better all on my own. When I came home, my wife had a wheelchair waiting for me. I said, "Honey! OUT! OUT! OUT!"

I had plans to get back in shape all by myself. I went upstairs, and I started to lift weights. It took one gigantic effort not to faint.

Then I went for a walk. I was walking along, and my mouth didn't want to work. That's when I realized I had a problem. I had a real problem. I knew that I needed to get more help.

It was about March 2012 when Alice reached out to Maura Silverman, a very well-known advocate in the aphasia community. That's when we got things started. I did work and work and work for her. She put me through hell, and I loved it.

That's when my progress really began. I could talk again and that made me happy!

Sometimes you have to make challenges fun! I made a little bet with myself. If I did what she wanted me to do, I could order a vanilla milkshake on my way home. But I didn't know how to say "vanilla milkshake."

I JUST DIDN'T WANT TO GIVE UP! I practiced, and I practiced, and I practiced. Maybe it took me four or five weeks. But I finally got it. "VANILLA MILKSHAKE!"

The Aphasia Center was the next stop. It was a six-week program. I went for six hours a day, five days a week for six weeks.

By the end of the week, I was exhausted—totally flat out exhausted! It was really hard work. Then again, I could speak a little bit better again.

So, Alice and I decided to move back to Wyomissing, Pennsylvania, and I began seeing Dr. Jeffrey Marrongelle—a doctor I have now been seeing for twenty-five years.

I also went to three other places to get help for the aphasia.

I have gone to twenty-one doctors and therapists in total. But I only ended up working with twelve. I have seen some really, really good doctors. I have seen some really, really bad doctors.

SOME DOCTORS WILL TELL YOU THAT YOU WON'T GET BETTER. I HAVE CHOSEN NOT TO BELIEVE THEM. I WILL GET BETTER! YOU HAVE TO BELIEVE IN YOURSELF!

After five years of hard work, I started to do the things that I really wanted to do.

I took singing and speaking lessons. I took horseback riding lessons at Rein and Shine. It was amazing. You sit up on a horse. Once you look one way, it goes that way. You look another way, and it will go in that direction.

Unbelievable!

I am taking CrossFit with my friends at Rhapsody CrossFit three days a week.

I am working on my right arm with Dr. Maysa Hannawi, who graduated from MUSC Physical Therapy.

I am taking two classes at the College of Charleston.

I never thought I would do these things before I had my stroke.

So then I had enough courage to reach out to someone to teach me how to speak. And that's when I found Rebecca Martin, a coach in California.

I didn't want to tell just one person at a time. I wanted to share my story with the world.

So, here I am!

I can't read the way I used to!

I can't speak the way I used to!

I can't write the way I used to!

BUT... I can read, speak, and write.

These are things I could not do eight years ago.

My leg has gotten better!

My arm is my friend!

I got my speech back... MAYBE eighty-five percent, but that's okay!

SO, I AM HERE TO GIVE THIS ADVICE:

NEVER, NEVER, NEVER GIVE UP!

KEEP YOUR EYE ON THE GOAL. YOU JUST HAVE TO FIND A WAY.

YOU CAN DO IT.

DO NOT LET ANYONE SAY TO YOU, "THAT'S NOT POSSIBLE."

IT IS POSSIBLE.

KEEP LOOKING, AND FIND YOUR OWN WAY!

HERE IS ONE MORE PIECE OF ADVICE:

Treat one person at a time.

I know that your days are full.

If you had a rough time with one of your patients, let go of it, AND COME TO ME!

Because I am one person. You have one hour to work with me. So work with me.

Don't let the past get in your way.

Don't let the future get in your way.

You have ONE person. ONE, ONE, ONE PERSON AT A TIME!

AND THAT PERSON IS ME!

TAKE THE OPPORTUNITY TO CHANGE A LIFE LIKE MINE!

THANK YOU!

HONORABLE MENTIONS

These friends, family members, therapists, and doctors all have a special place in Jeffrey's heart. Without them, he wouldn't be where he is today.

Dr. Jeffrey Marrongelle:
- Dr. Marrongelle has served an instrumental role in Jeffrey's recovery. Having been Jeffrey's doctor since 1985, he has been there through everything down to the most unbelievable developments. After Jeffrey's stroke, Dr. Marrongelle was able to strengthen his vocal cords and challenged what was deemed impossible. Jeffrey saw him every week for two and a half years. Now, Jeffrey visits him once every four months.

Stiche Center:
- Immediately following his stroke and discharge from the hospital where his stroke happened, Jeffrey went to the Stiche Center in Winston-Salem, North Carolina. According to Jeffrey, this was the most amazing hospital where he regained much hope.

The Aphasia Center:
- Working with Dr. Lori Bartles-Tobin at the Aphasia Center for five straight days over a six-day period, Jeffrey began to notice progress in his speech. Dr. Bartles-Tobin was a hoot and was able to help Jeffrey get to the point where he was comfortable teaching again up to a certain degree.

Professor Scott Nice:

- As a professor of voice and movement at the University of North Carolina-Wilmington, Professor Nice worked with Jeffrey for four months. Together, they "shook things out." To Jeffrey's surprise, the new movement helped greatly.

Lingraphica Incorporated:

- Jeffrey met with his group of doctors, lawyers, and real estate agents every other week for two years. This mismatched band of twenty people bonded over their shared experiences with aphasia. Through their struggles and triumphs, these everyday community members helped each other reclaim parts of their lives.

The Moss Center:

- Jeffrey went to Karen Mohen's speech class every week for two years. With a small group of twelve people from all walks of life, this tight-knit community worked through hard things together, guided by their amazing teacher.

McKinley Pollard:

- Working with Front & Center Marketing while a senior at the College of Charleston, McKinley has been on this journey with Jeffrey to write this book for a year. Jeffrey has been blown away by her ability to stay on track and manage so many things at once. As a full-time student, president of multiple clubs and honor societies, and a Martin Scholar with two internships, Jeffrey can't keep up with her, but he certainly tries. McKinley is also next to Jeffrey at Rhapsody Fitness tackling tough workouts. Upon first meeting McKinley, Jeffrey knew it would be difficult to get to know her. He found that she was always listening attentively. According to Jeffrey, she's one of the most interesting people, who is beautiful inside and out. Jeffrey is proud that he could bring out her true smile often.

Trinity Wheeler:
- After about two years at Rhapsody Fitness, Jeffrey and Alice really got to know the cofounder of this special gym. As a Broadway producer, Trinity is always putting on a show and is quite personable. Working together on the short film *Rhapsody Presents: The Fishers* with Matchlight, Jeffrey, Alice, and Trinity have formed a special bond that ultimately played out on the big screen.

Grace Privette Farren:
- After hearing about Grace through a Rhapsody friend, Jeffrey started working with her as his speech pathologist. Despite being well into her retirement, Grace was happy to help. Jeffrey's biggest challenge and accomplishment was memorizing the Gettysburg Address. It took eight months of hard work, but he finally got it down. Jeffrey has been working with Grace for a year.

Keith Schmehl:
- Meeting at Peirce Junior College, Jeffrey and Keith became very close friends. They went through a lot

together, and Keith has been a constant in Jeffrey's life as a very supportive and kind friend.

SPECIAL THANKS TO

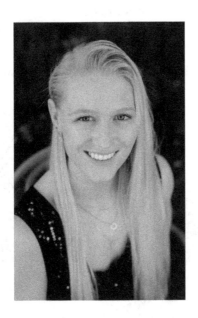

MCKINLEY POLLARD

Born in Roanoke, Virginia, McKinley ventured to Charleston for higher education where she is finishing up her senior year at the College of Charleston. A Martin Scholar and Charleston Wine + Food Marketing Fellow, McKinley is a leader on campus as the president of the CofC Women's Club Soccer Team, president of the American Marketing Association, president of Lambda Pi Eta, member of the National Society of Leadership and Success, and an alumna of Delta Gamma.

Complementing her studies with hands-on experience, she is a client relations and marketing manager for a national staff outsourcing firm called PFP Logistics and special projects coordinator for Front & Center, a woman-owned-and-operated branding and marketing firm serving entrepreneurs and small business owners from coast to coast.

When she is not hard at work, you may find McKinley chewing on a barbell at Rhapsody Fitness, searching for an adrenaline rush, or finding the next foodie haven.

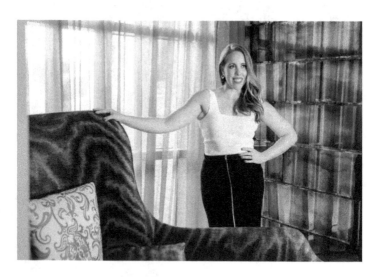

FRONT & CENTER

Based in Charleston, South Carolina, Front & Center is a bespoke business coaching, brand development, and marketing firm exclusively serving small businesses and entrepreneurs across the country.

Founded by Mary Beth Henderson in 2016, Front & Center is committed to reputation before recognition in its mission to empower you to live a life you love on your terms through your venture.

The Front & Center team was proud to help Jeffery put pen to paper for his incredible story and bring his publication to fruition in collaboration with Bublish, Inc.

Learn more about Front & Center online at www.frontandcenterllc.com.